# Real Tips for Pregnancy

How to Best Deal with the Prenatal and
Postnatal Period: Nutrition, Fitness and a
Home Workout Plan for Pregnant Women

*Claire Blanchard*

ISBN Paperback: 978-1-80157-220-0

Printed by IngramSpark

First printing edition 2021.
.

# Table of Content

# Introduction

Getting pregnant and childbirth are two of life's greatest miracles.

Most women, when asked the question, "What was the most memorable event in your life?" often cite pregnancy and childbirth.

It's like a gift from above. There is just no denying the powerful emotions that pregnancy and childbirth can create in parents.

However, while pregnancy is glorious and a rewarding experience, the hard truth is that there is a nutrition and fitness aspect that cannot be neglected.

There is also a flip side to this shiny coin. Many women often end up feeling that pregnancy has ruined their shapely figure and the stretch marks have disfigured them.

They automatically assume that once they've given birth, their bodies will never go back to the shape they originally used to be. Weight gain, stretch marks, a loss of sex appeal, etc. are negative consequences that women consider a trade-off to having a bouncy little baby.

Nothing could be further from the truth.

Yes... pregnancy will result in weight gain. This is only natural and in fact, it's healthy. However, the weight gain can be maintained without letting it get out of control.

All weight that is gained during pregnancy can be lost after pregnancy. After all, it's just fat and the principles of fat loss are set in stone regardless if it's a pregnant woman or an obese man.

It will take you time to shed the fat... but there is no hurry. Slow and steady wins the race. With patience and persistence, you can definitely lose the excess fat after childbirth.

If you persist, you can even get fitter and be in better shape after childbirth than you were previously. Your body is a marvelous organism and it will adapt to whatever demands you place upon it.

What truly matters is that you believe that it can be achieved. You must release any false beliefs that pregnancy and childbirth will result in you becoming an overweight, dumpy or unattractive woman.

The natural state of things will mean that you gain weight during pregnancy and you'll lose it all after childbirth.

Even the world's most female celebrities have had the following things to say about pregnancy and weight gain.

*"You have to eat to feed your baby. And I have a girl, so I want her to see some day why her mom has good self-esteem and good body issues. It gets you down sometimes, I'm not going to lie. I've had days where I'm like, 'Ugh, I wish this was easier.' But it's not, and that's OK."* – **Jennifer Love Hewitt**

*"I'm taking it week-by-week so I don't get frustrated with myself. If I had a long-term goal and that's all I thought about, I think it would set me back more."* – **Jessica Simpson**

*"I think if you ask any pregnant mom, they're like 'I want my body back. But it takes time. It takes nine months for your body to get that way, and it's putting on that weight on purpose. The second I start to get down like, 'What happened to my body?' I look at my beautiful baby—and I've never been more appreciative for this body that I have."* – **Hillary Duff**

The point to take away from all this is that it is normal to gain weight and it takes time to lose it. Will you feel down and depressed now and again?

Yes, you will. But you will persist and ultimately, you will get the body you desire.

There is much more to just losing weight after childbirth. You'll also need to know how to eat right during your pregnancy, how
 to do certain exercises to stay fit and strong, what types of supplements to use, etc.

This book will give you helpful tips and techniques that you can use to get healthy and stay n shape during and after your pregnancy.

Do note that this is all just advice. It will only work if you adhere and apply the information within this book to your life.

You ready?

Happy Reading!

# Pre-conception: What you need to know!

Before even getting pregnant, you should be aware that your health, habits, diet, fitness level and many other factors will directly or indirectly affect your pregnancy and the fetal development.

One example would be pregnant women who have the smoking habit. This does a lot of damage to both the mother and the child within.

If you're going to get pregnant, you should eliminate all your negative habits prior to conception.

Ideally, you should exercise more, eat a clean diet, avoid alcohol and smoking is a definite no-no. If you have any issues with substance abuse, etc. you should eliminate all these before planning to have a baby.

Proper nutrition is crucial in the stages of pre-conception and during pregnancy.

The beautiful baby in your belly is physically incapable of providing for itself. All the food and nutrition it gets is determined by you. Surely you want nothing but the best for your baby.

A fetus also does not display any visible signs of malnourishment during your monthly check-ups. That means, even your doctor will not be able to ascertain if the baby is getting all the nutrients it needs.

Therefore, you will have to ensure that you're eating enough for two and getting all the necessary vitamins and nutrients. Only by being proactive and taking an active interest in your nutrition will you be able to keep both the baby and yourself healthy and happy.

Here are a few tips if you're in the pre-conception stage.

- **No smoking & no alcohol**

No negotiation here.

- **Consume 400 to 800 micrograms (400 to 800 mcg or 0.4 to 0.8 mg) of folic acid daily.**

  You should speak to your doctor about this. He/she will be able to guide you in this matter. Folic acid reduces the risk of birth defects related to the spine and brain.

- **Get your other health problems under control**

  If you're diabetic, obese, have asthma, etc. you should get all these problems under control first before getting pregnant. All these health issues may cause pregnancy complications.

- **Get fit and healthy**

  Exercise more. Build up your strength and stamina.

  When you're pregnant, it will be easier on your body if you're strong and healthy.

- **Ask your partner to play an active role**

If your partner smokes or engages in detrimental activities, they should try and quit for the sake of the baby.

At the very least, if they can't quit, they shouldn't smoke around you or tempt you by consuming alcohol around you.

# Nutrition and the Best Foods to Eat During Pregnancy

The ancient Greek physician, Hippocrates, once said, "Let food be thy medicine and let medicine be thy food."

This definitely holds true when you're pregnant. A clean, healthy and wholesome diet will work wonders for you and your baby.

We live in a society that is smothered with a plethora of food choices. The hard truth is that the majority of these foods are detrimental to our bodies in the long run.

Additives, preservatives, chemicals, processed foods, junk foods, genetically modified foods, etc. are all part of our diet these days and are wreaking havoc on our health.

 Obesity has become an epidemic. The numbers of people suffering from diabetes, high cholesterol, digestive issues, etc. have skyrocketed. The main culprit – our diet.

Changing one's diet and eating clean is a Herculean task. You absolutely can't do it overnight and don't even think that will- power will work.

You will need to make small changes to your diet gradually till you form the habits of eating right. That is why, it is imperative that you start making these changes 3 months before getting pregnant.

You'll then be able to ease into a healthy diet relatively smoothly and easily.

## How many calories should I consume?

Many women wonder about this. They do not want to consume too many calories for fear of putting on weight... but then they
 have all these sudden food cravings that seemed to pop out of nowhere.

The first thing you should note – Do NOT obsess over your

calories when you're pregnant. Now is really not the time to be analyzing and counting your calories.

Pregnancy gives you the permission to take 9 months off from the calorie counting and agonizing over the numbers. That being said, it's also not a free pass to gorge yourself on whatever food comes your way.

Eat sufficient food but eat the proper food. Restricting your calories could potentially harm your baby.

Low birth weight, poor fetal development, weakness in the mother, etc. are all often related to not consuming enough food. Always remember, whatever weight you gain can be burnt off after childbirth.

**A warning though** – If you consume too many calories there are problems too. You will gain too much weight which will put you at risk for diabetes, heart problems, early labor, pre- eclamsia, etc.

It's all about balance. Eat enough for both you and your baby. Eat healthy and eat in moderation.

Before going any further, you will need to calculate your pre- pregnancy Recommended Daily Caloric Intake. This is actually just your normal caloric requirement if you were not pregnant.

You can find this out at http://www.freedieting.com/tools/c alorie_calculator.htm

Now we'll look at the foods that you should be consuming during your pregnancy. Truth be told, healthy foods are healthy foods whether you are pregnant or not. It doesn't matter if you're male female, young or old... Good food choices are always beneficial.

The only difference is that now, you're pregnant and it's even more important to eat right because another life depends and is affected by your food choices. Yup... the pressure is on.

## Foods You Must Eat

In the fitness industry, there is a saying, "Calories are not created equal."

That means, you could eat 300 calories from different foods and have a world of different results. For example, if you ate 2 bananas and 2 apples a day, which would roughly be 300 calories. What if you got all 300 calories from 2 scoops of chocolate ice cream?

Would the benefits be the same? Guess which one is going to be better for your baby?

## 1. Eat whole foods

Whole foods could also be called single ingredient foods. For example, a broccoli is a single ingredient food.

You pick it up... you know what it is... and you know it grew from the ground.

Now let's look at white bread?

Most people have no idea how it was made, what ingredients were used... and how in the world did they get the bread so white, anyway?

The moment you have no idea what goes into the food, it's best you avoid it. White bread uses refined flour that is bleached white and all kinds of artificial ingredients go into making a loaf.

None of it is doing your body any favors. Avoid processed foods and stick to natural foods.

**2. Eat fruits and veggies** This is common sense. We all know that fruits and vegetables contain a ton of vitamins and minerals that do us good. Be consistent with your diet. You must eat these daily.

An apple a day keeps the doctor away.

You can't eat 7 apples on Saturday and expect to get the job done. It doesn't work that way. Consistency is key.

**3. Make sure you're only eating good carbs**

Carbs have received a bad reputation over the years. The truth is that carbs are essential for us. This is especially so when you're pregnant. Carbs give you energy and make up a sizeable chunk of your required calories.
What matters is that you consume carbs from healthy sources. Fruits vegetables, whole grain breads, potatoes, oats, quinoa, brown rice, etc. are all excellent carb sources.

Pizzas, white bread, white flour products,

etc. are bad carbs that should be avoided.

## 4. Eat enough protein

These are essential too. Get your proteins from lean meats, eggs, beef and beans. Once again, focus on the "single ingredient" requirement. A few cuts of lean chicken breast are good. A chicken nugget is NOT good. A slab of steak is good. A few sausages are NOT good.

## 5. Try and keep it organic if possible.

While this can be a little costly, it is highly beneficial. If you can afford to eat organic for the 9 months that you're pregnant, go for it.

Organic foods are free of pesticides or synthetic fertilizers.

In the event that your budget does not allow you to go completely organic, then make sure some of the foods that you consume are organic.

Foods such as apples, bell peppers, celery, cherries, grapes, nectarines, peaches, pears, potatoes, raspberries, spinach and strawberries have been found to contain high levels of pesticides. So, try and keep these organic, if you can.

## 6. Eat the right kind of fat

Extra virgin olive oil and virgin coconut oil are two of the best types of fat you can consume. In fact, of the two, the coconut oil is better.

Saturated fats are found in meat and animal products such as butter. These are best eaten in moderation.

If you forget everything mentioned earlier in this chapter and just print out and follow the food list below, you will do just fine.

| *Vitamin* | *Food Source* |
|---|---|
| Vitamin A | Liver, carrots, sweet potatoes, kale, spinach, collard greens, cantaloupe, eggs, mangos and peas |
| Vitamin B6 | Fortified cereals, bananas, baked potatoes, watermelon, chick peas and chicken breast |
| Vitamin B12 | Red meat, poultry, fish, shellfish, eggs and dairy foods |
| Vitamin C | Citrus fruits, raspberries, bell peppers, green beans, strawberries, papaya, potatoes, broccoli and tomatoes |
| Calcium | Dairy products, fortified juices, fortified butters and fortified cereals, spinach, broccoli, okra, sweet potatoes, lentils, tofu, Chinese cabbage, kale and broccoli. |

| | |
|---|---|
| Vitamin D | Milk, fortified cereals, eggs and fatty fish (salmon, catfish and mackerel) |
| Vitamin E | Vegetable oil, wheat germ, nuts, spinach and fortified cereal |

24|

| | |
|---|---|
| Folic Acid | Oranges, orange juice, strawberries, leafy vegetables, spinach, beets, broccoli, cauliflower, peas, pasta, beans, nuts and sunflower seeds |
| Iron | Red meat and poultry, legumes, vegetables, some grains and fortified cereals |
| Niacin (Vitamin B3) | Eggs, meats, fish, peanuts, whole grains, bread products, fortified cereals and milk |
| Protein | Beans, poultry, red meat, fish, shellfish, eggs, milk, cheese, tofu, yogurt, fortified cereal and protein bars |

| | |
|---|---|
| Riboflavin (Vitamin B2) | Whole grains, dairy products, red meat, pork, poultry, fish, fortified cereals and eggs |
| Thiamin (Vitamin B1) | Whole grains, pork, fortified cereals, wheat germ and eggs |
| Zinc | Red meats, poultry, beans, nuts, grains, oysters, dairy products and fortified cereals |

# Supplements Before & During Pregnancy

Besides food, your body will also require supplements. It is extremely difficult to get all the necessary nutrients, vitamins and minerals that your body needs from food alone.

Your diet will have to be varied and your knowledge of nutrition will have to be good to get a completely balanced diet with no deficiencies.

Most women just do not have the time to watch their diet like a hawk and note the different vitamins they're getting. By consuming supplements, you'll be able to pick up the slack from a diet that is deficient in a few vitamins and minerals.

Some basic knowledge would be very helpful though. When you understand what you're eating, how much you should eat, why
 you're eating it... pregnancy nutrition will be much easier to get right.

There is a list further down with 14 important supplements you should consume. Do note that the Recommended Daily Allowances are just a rough estimate. Speak to your doctor and tailor your supplement intake to best suit your needs.

Another point you should be aware of is that there are negative consequences of overdosing on specific vitamins. This usually occurs from eating foods that contain a certain vitamin and consuming supplements which contain that vitamin too. Now there is a surplus in your body.

This is why it's important to tell your doctor during your prenatal appointments what you're eating and what vitamins, medications and supplements (including herbal) you're taking too.

This will help them to assess your diet. Do not leave any details out regardless of how insignificant you may believe them to be.
 These are the supplements that you will need.

# 1. Vitamin A

Vitamin A is crucial for the development of the baby's bones, teeth, heart, ears, eyes and immune system.

Aim to consume at least 770 micrograms (or 2565 IU, as it is labeled on nutritional labels) of Vitamin A per day. This will double when nursing to 1300 micrograms (4,330 IU).

Overdosing on Vitamin A can cause birth defects and liver toxicity. **Do NOT consume more than 3000 mcg (10,000 IU) per day.**

Vitamin A can be found in liver, carrots, sweet potatoes, kale spinach collard greens, cantaloupe, eggs, mangos and peas.

## 2. Vitamin B6

This vitamin which is also known as Pyridoxine helps with the development of the baby's brain and nervous system. It also encourages the growth of new red blood cells in both mom and baby. Some women report that B6 has helped to alleviate their morning sickness.

Pregnant women should consume at least 1.9 mg per day of Vitamin B6. That amount rises slightly when nursing to 2.0 mg per day.

Vitamin B6 can be found in fortified cereals, as well as bananas, baked potatoes, watermelon, chick peas and chicken breast.

### 3. Vitamin B12

Vitamin B12 works together with folic acid to help aid in the production of healthy red blood cells and promotes development of a healthy brain and nervous system in the baby.
 The body usually has sufficient stores of B12 and it's very rare to have a B12 deficiency.

Pregnant women should consume at least 2.6 mcg (104 IU) of B12per day, nursing mothers 2.8 mcg (112 IU).

It can found in red meat, poultry, fish, shellfish, eggs and dairy foods.

## 4. Vitamin C

Probably the most famous of all the vitamins, Vitamin C will help both mommy and baby to absorb iron and build a healthy immune system. Other than that, it will hold the cells together and help the body to build tissue.

Pregnant women should consume at least 80-85 mg of Vitamin C per day, nursing mothers no less than 120 mg per day.

Vitamin C can be found in citrus fruits, raspberries, bell peppers, green beans, strawberries, papaya, potatoes, broccoli and tomatoes, as well as in many cough drops and other supplements.

## 5. Calcium

This vitamin is crucial for building your baby's bones and promotes optimal functioning of the baby's brain and heart.

Pregnant women should consume at least 1200 mg of calcium a day, nursing mothers 1000 mg per day.

Calcium can be found in dairy products, such as milk, cheese, yoghurt and, to a lesser extent, ice cream, as well as fortified juices, butters and cereals, spinach, broccoli, okra, sweet potatoes, lentils, tofu, Chinese cabbage, kale and broccoli. It is also widely available in supplement form.

## 6. Vitamin D

Vitamin D aids in the absorption of calcium. This will lead to healthy bones in both mother and child.

Women who are pregnant or nursing should consume at least 2000 IU of Vitamin D per day.

Babies usually require more Vitamin D than adults. Your doctor may recommend a Vitamin D supplement and baby formula is also fortified with Vitamin D.

Vitamin D is rarely found in sufficient amounts in ordinary foods. It can, however, be found in milk (most milk is fortified) as well as fortified cereals, eggs and fatty fish like salmon, catfish and mackerel. Vitamin D is also found in sunshine, so women and children found to have a mild Vitamin D deficiency may be told to spend more time in the sun.

### 7. Vitamin E

Vitamin E helps the baby's body to form and use its muscles and red blood cells.

Pregnant women should consume at least 20 mg of Vitamin E per day but not more than 540 mg.

Vitamin E can be found in naturally in vegetable oil, wheat germ, nuts, spinach and fortified cereals as well as in supplemental form.

It's better to get your Vitamin E from natural food sources than synthetic supplements.

### 8. Folic Acid

This is one of the most important vitamins during pregnancy and is vital for the development of a healthy baby. The body uses Folic Acid for the replication of DNA, cell growth and tissue formation.

Folic acid deficiencies result in many nasty

birth defects such as spina bifida (a condition in which the spinal cord does not form completely), anencephaly (underdevelopment of the brain) and encephalocele (a condition in which brain tissue protrudes out to the skin from an abnormal opening in the skull).

All of these conditions occur during the first 28 days of fetal development, usually before the mother even knows she's pregnant.

It's imperative that you get enough folic acid in your diet prior to getting pregnant.

Pregnant woman should consume at least 0.6-0.8 mg of Folic Acid per day.

Folic Acid can be found in oranges, orange juice, strawberries, leafy vegetables, spinach, beets, broccoli, cauliflower, peas, pasta, beans, nuts and sunflower seeds, as well as in supplements and fortified cereals.

### 9. Iron

This is another important vitamin that helps with cell development, blood cell formation and placenta formation.

Women who are pregnant should have at least 27 mg of iron per day.

Iron can be found in red meat and poultry, legumes, vegetables, some grains and fortified cereals.

## 10.    Niacin

This is known as Vitamin B3 and helps to keep the mother's digestive system functioning optimally as well as gives the baby energy to develop well.

Pregnant women should have an intake of at least 18 mg of Niacin per day.
 Niacin can be found in foods that are high in protein, such as eggs, meats, fish and peanuts, as well as whole grains, bread products, fortified cereals and milk.

## 11.    Protein

Protein is the building block of the body's cells. All growth and development of the body requires protein and protein is especially important in the second and third trimester, when both Mom and baby are growing the fastest.

Pregnant and nursing women should consume at least 70g of protein per day, which is about 25g more than the average women needs before pregnancy.

Protein can be found naturally in beans, poultry, red meats, fish, shellfish, eggs, milk, cheese, tofu and yogurt. It is also available in supplements, fortified cereals and protein bars.

## 12.   Riboflavin

This is also known as Vitamin B2. It gives the body energy and helps in the development of the baby's bones, muscles and nervous system.

Pregnant women should consume at least 1.4 mg of Riboflavin per day, nursing mothers 1.6 mg.

Riboflavin can be found in whole grains, dairy products, red meat, pork and poultry, fish, fortified cereals and eggs.

## 13.    Thiamin

Thiamin is Vitamin B1 assists in the development of the baby's organs and central nervous system.

Pregnant women and nursing mothers should consume at least

1.4 mg of Thiamin a day.

Thiamin can be found in whole grain foods, pork, fortified cereals, wheat germ and eggs.

## 14.    Zinc

Zinc is vital for the growth of your fetus because it aids in cell division, the primary process in the growth of baby's tiny tissues and organs. It also helps Mom and baby to produce insulin and other enzymes.

Pregnant women should have an intake of at least 11-12 mg of Zinc per day.

Zinc can be found naturally in red meats, poultry, beans, nuts, grains, oysters and dairy products, as well as fortified cereals and supplements.

# Nutrition & Fitness during Your Pregnancy

This chapter will breakdown the nutrition and exercise depending on each trimester.

By now, you should be aware of what foods to consume and you should realize that it helps to stay active during your pregnancy.

So, this chapter will be more about taking action and

implementing the nutrition information provided earlier. You'll also be told what exercises to do to help you.

## The First Trimester – Nutrition & Exercise Tips

### Nutrition

During your first trimester, your calorie intake does not have to significantly increase. However, you must ensure that you're
getting all the right vitamins, minerals, etc. This is especially true for folic acid.

You should NOT be dieting or trying to keep your weight down. It is normal to gain some weight during your first trimester. Enjoy the pregnancy process.

Do not fight it for vanity reasons.

## Exercise

Your strength and stamina prior to getting pregnant will determine how much exercise you can do during your first trimester.

There is a fallacy that pregnant women should not exercise for fear of injuring their baby. This is not true. Pregnancy is not an excuse to become a couch potato.
 In fact, your pregnancy will be easier if you're moderately active. The key word here is **moderately**.

Avoid all high impact training regimens such as HIIT, Crossfit or Tabata during your first trimester.

One of the best forms of exercise that you can do is brisk walking. In fact, just going for a daily 30 minute walk can be highly beneficial. Ask your partner to follow you too so that you have company and there is some bonding time.

If you were highly active before your pregnancy, you may miss your cardio sessions.

You may still engage in cardio sessions as long as they are low impact. A stationary bike is a good way to break a sweat.

Swimming is also excellent. It is low impact and yet, very effective.

High impact exercises such as kickboxing, skipping, full body workouts, etc. should be avoided.

Do not workout to the point where you are breathless and gasping for air. Your goal is to be active... You're not training for the Olympics.

You want to exercise to get your blood circulation and your heart pumping. It's more about activity than achievement. Avoid strenuous workouts.

# The Second Trimester – Nutrition & Exercise Tips

## Nutrition

As far as what you're supposed to eat, the food choices will be the same for all 3 trimesters. The only difference is that the calories will vary.

As you go into your second and third trimester you should increase your daily caloric intake by 300 calories.

This will help to compensate for the increasing rate of your baby's growth. If your pre-pregnancy caloric intake was 1800 calories you should consume 2100 calories a day.

If it was 1400 calories you should consume 1700 calories, and so on and so forth.

Will you gain weight? Yes, definitely.

Is that ok? You bet it is. <u>Now is not the time to worry about losing weight.</u>

In fact, it is healthy to gain some weight during pregnancy. Eat the correct foods and eat more so that there are sufficient calories and nutrients in your body for both you and your baby.

## Exercise

Unlike the first trimester, most women do not experience morning sickness or fatigue. The body has adapted to the pregnancy and usually, that means more energy.

You should probably feel like you have more energy in your second trimester.

That will mean that you can be more active. Of course, the same rule applies about low impact exercises. However, now you should aim to incorporate strength training exercises in your regimen.

Pay more attention to exercises that tone your back muscles, neck muscles and legs. Pregnancy will place some strain on all these muscles. You often hear of pregnant women complaining that their backs, necks and legs ache or feel tired. Now you know why.

These are some of the best strength exercises that you can do during your second trimester. If you do not know how

to do them, you can always Google them or
look them up on YouTube.

- Squats
- Step ups
- Lunges
- Modified side planks (knees at 90
  degrees on ground)
- Bird dog
- Bicep/triceps curls
- Straight Leg calf stretch
- Hip flexor stretch

As far as cardio goes, you may carry on
with your walking or stationary bike
workouts sessions.

The thing about exercise is that it
really depends on the individual.

There are women who are extremely
sporty before pregnancy and can go
running or even play sports during
pregnancy.

Is this advisable? It depends. Only
you will know your own capabilities.

Ideally, contact sports should be avoided.

The best person to speak to, will be your doctor. He/she will be able to advise you on the best types of exercises that are best suited for you.

Generally, most women will do just fine walking or doing a stationary bike. There is really no need to overdo it or try and prove that pregnancy is not holding you back.

Also, do not exercise more than you have to just because you're consuming more calories during your second trimester and you want to burn them off and stay slim. This is counter-productive and will affect both you and the baby adversely.

Enjoy your pregnancy. You will have the happy glow of a pregnant woman. There is no need to worry about looking like a Swimsuit Illustrated model.

## The Third Trimester – Nutrition & Exercise Tips Nutrition

By now, you should have had several appointments with your doctor and he/she should be monitoring your progress.

What your calorie requirement should be in the third trimester will be determined by your condition. Your doctor will advise you if you need to eat more or less. Just follow the doctor's advice.

## Exercise

By now, the baby bump should be showing significantly. It may hinder most of the exercise movements that you're accustomed too. However, you will still be able to go walking or use the stationary bike.

The goal is just to be moving. Don't focus on sweating or getting your heart pumping. It's not about intensity. It's about movement.

You can follow the same strength training exercises mentioned during the second trimester.

Alternatively, you may wish to go for a few classes of yoga specifically designed for pregnant women. These classes often focus on stretching and also relieving the tension in the back, legs and neck area.

In the last trimester, every movement might be an effort. If you feel like you're not in the mood to exercise or it's just too much effort, you may take a break.

Being happy also matters because if you're happy, the baby will be happy too.

You may also wish to meditate and relax to clear your mind and de-stress. There is immense power in mediation.

# The Baby has arrived! What now?

This is the part where you cuddle your baby and make cooing

noises. It's also the part where you order your partner to do your every bidding because you're recovering.

After childbirth, you may slowly reduce your calorie consumption. Carry on with your clean eating and eat sufficient quantities of nutritious food.

You will be lactating and will need to breastfeed your child. Once again, the best person to speak to, will be your doctor.

Generally, there are a few breastfeeding tips you should be aware of.

- It will hurt initially
- Moisturize your nipples with olive oil
- Use comfortable bras
- Drink lots of water and stay hydrated at all times
- Eat well and consume sufficient calories

# What next?

There will be many other things to do as a new mommy. You can learn all these from a guide for new mothers.

Those are beyond the scope of this book which is focused more on nutrition and fitness.

Which brings us to the next point... getting your body back in shape after childbirth.

2 or 3 weeks after you have given birth; you will be ready to start on your exercise program.

Now... and only NOW... do you start focusing on attaining your dream body. Of course, before you can get there, you will need to shed the weight.

Once again you will check your daily caloric requirement. Once you have a number, you will aim for a 500 calorie deficit daily. This is a safe number to aim for.

Don't aim to cut your calories too low. This does not speed up your results. It will just plateau your body and impede any further progress.

Now that you've given birth, you can exercise often. However there are a few things you must be aware of.

It takes six weeks to three months for your body to heal after pregnancy.

What that means is that your training program should still be low impact. Forget HIIT training or sprinting. Low impact training is your mantra.

Don't worry. You will still lose weight at a steady rate. As long as your body is at a caloric deficit, it is inevitable that you lose weight.

If you went walking twice a day with each session lasting 30 to 45 minutes, you will be amazed at how much weight you will lose.

Want to challenge yourself? Walk uphill. Want more challenge? Add ankle weights and walk.

That's how you do it.

As long as your diet is clean and healthy and you're at a daily caloric deficit... you will lose the weight.

Many women get impatient and want fast results. Weight loss is not a fast process. It doesn't matter if you're pregnant or not... Losing weight is an uphill task that takes time.

Never give up on it just because you think it will take you 8

months to lose all the weight you've gained. The time is going to pass anyway.

8 months later, you will still be where you are if you don't make an active effort to change.

So, keep at it slowly but surely. Take a photo on day one and take a photo 6 months later. You will be blown away by the results.
Most women are able to return to their pre-pregnancy body shape within six months, just by doing low impact cardio daily and maintaining a caloric deficit.
If they can do it, so can you.

# Taking Your Fitness to the Next Level

After 6 months, see your doctor and check if you're able to increase the intensity of your training program.

Once you get the green light, it's time to pull out all the stops.

Start training with weights and combine your resistance training with cardio sessions.

Keep your cardio sessions short but at a high-intensity. This will put your body in fat burning mode for hours.

The principles are the same. A caloric deficit and training.

To go from moderately fit to super fit is just a matter of intensity and time.

The more intensely you train the better your results will be. Train intensely for 3 months and that will be good... but spend a year training and your body will be fantastic. The longer the duration, the better your body.

Mindset is also important.

The birth of a child does not doom you to living life with an out- of-shape body. It's not a lifelong curse of being fat.

In fact, there is nothing stopping you from getting the body that you want. The only thing stopping you, is you.

Now you are a mother and you have every reason to be a living example for your child. Set a fitness goal for yourself.

Strive towards it. Stay focused and set small, measurable goals. Be happy with the little achievements and celebrate them. The end goal is a result of all the milestones you reached along the way.

Time flies, and before you know it, you will have the body your heart desires. You will be the envy of the other women.

They'll probably think you have good genetics or that you did liposuction. People often put others down to lift themselves up. It helps them see past their own failings.

You, however, will know better. You will know that it took effort, discipline and determination. Aren't these the qualities you want your child to have?

Of course you do. They will learn more by watching what you do rather than by listening to what you say. Be an example for them. They'll be proud of you... and more importantly, you'll be a proud mommy... and proud of mommy too.

That is truly priceless.

**"Feeling fat lasts nine months...
but the joy of
being a mom
lasts forever."**

# Keeping Fit: A Route to Sanity

In a world where many people act based on what they see, it is vital to focus on both the outward and inward aspects of your life. Many people will judge you based on your appearance. In fact, some people of the opposite sex can turn you down because they feel you aren't sexy enough for them.

Indeed, it is not ideal to judge people only based on their physical appearance. Nonetheless, you need to realize that we aren't living in an ideal world. So, while developing your intellect and emotional strength, you'll do yourself a lot of good by also investing in your physical appearance. Some people will never give you the chance to show what you can do because of the way you look.

Therefore, it is critical to improve your physique. Besides, the insensitive comments you can get, especially on social media because of your body shape, can be depressing. Therefore, keeping
fit is a route to sanity in the modern world. This

chapter will explore what a workout plan is and the link between your physical and mental health.

## What is a Home Workout Plan?

Indeed, we cannot deny the added advantages of visiting a gym or hiring a physical trainer to develop your physique. An expert has both the knowledge and experience to give you a customized routine that will get the requisite results. Nonetheless, you don't need a gym membership to build your muscle or lose weight.

If you've been observant enough, you'll notice that many people post pictures and videos about their home workout routines online. It is true that you shouldn't believe everything you see on the internet because many people post false information just to get likes and positive remarks. Nevertheless, the reality is that many people are improving their physical appearance without leaving their homes. You can be one such person if you're ready to pay the price.

A home workout plan is a deliberately

structured routine to improve your physical appearance by carrying out various

exercises. Indeed, there are equipment and facilities that can make this process easier. Nonetheless, you don't have to break the bank to get a good sweat, lose weight, or develop your muscles. You can still lose weight or build your abs with minimal or no investment by choosing the right plan and tasks.

# Vital Features of an Effective Home Workout Plan

Just like any activity, there are vital components that are integral to the success of your home workout plan. Once these features are missing, you'll only have a plan but will never execute it. They include:

## Purpose

When you fail to define the reason for an activity, it will eventually become redundant. You need to ask yourself why you need to start regular exercises. Do you want to start so that you can post a picture on your social media profile? Do you want to do it because it is the current trend? If your reason is flimsy, you'll stop very soon.

Therefore, you have to ensure that you have a clearly defined objective before starting your plan. Endeavor to write your targets down so that you can tailor your plans in the right direction. Your goals will also help you to develop an effective diet plan that will support your commitment to physical activity.

## Vision

A vision is something you see long before it happens. Having a clear vision about the kind of person you want to be determines the kind of commitment you'll have today. It enables you to channel your energy and resources in the right direction.

The purpose of starting a workout will affect your vision. Meanwhile, your vision will determine the kind of exercises you'll perform. For example, if you're doing exercise to develop your abs, you'll not have a workout plan that encourages the development of butt muscles. The kind of physique you imagine yourself having is what will determine your routine.

## Gradual Process

Nothing you do in a hurry can stand the test of time. Rushing may earn you some quick results, but you'll not be able to sustain it.

Besides, impatience often leads to desperation, which often leads to disastrous outcomes. In the context of physical activities, it can make you engage in strenuous routines that can have adverse effects on your health.

You must never forget that developing your physique is a gradual process. Impatience and desperation can make you injure yourself or become discouraged along the way. You need to enjoy the process to make your home workout plan a success. It is good to use the body shape of others as inspiration, but you must never forget that it took them time to achieve that physique.

## Motivation

The fuel of any aspiration is passion. Zeal spurs you to follow up on a plan or strategy to ensure that you succeed. Your home workout plan will never become a reality when you lack motivation. You must be excited to do your press-ups every day.

Once you lose the desire to go on, you'll quit. So, use your vision as a springboard to get going, especially during days when you're tired or in a bad mood. Joining a fitness club may encourage you to sustain your momentum. Nonetheless, if you're self-motivated, you can still be consistent all by yourself.

**Commitment**

You cannot separate motivation and commitment. When you're motivated to carry out a task, you'll commit to it. A plan that lacks commitment will only remain on paper but will never be executed. Laziness is one of those factors that can stop you from achieving your desired body shape. So, ensure that you don't allow laxity and boredom to set it. Anyone can start working out, but only committed people can sustain the momentum in the long run. There are some critical tips that can help you sustain your plan. You'll learn about them in subsequent chapters.

# Link Between Physical Health and Mental Health

It is impossible to separate physical health from mental health because one affects the other. In other words, if you have poor physical health, it will affect you mentally. For example, if you're battling a chronic disease, it could lead to depression. In the same way, your mental health can also affect your physical health. For instance, if you're battling depression and anxiety, it could affect your eating habit and exercise.

Meanwhile, you cannot maintain your physical health if you have bad eating habits and don't exercise. Moreover, the definition of health, according to the World Health Organization, shows that both physical and psychological health must be constant before you can term a person as "healthy." Besides, social wellbeing is also a key part of overall health.

The following are ways your mental and physical health are interconnected:

**Depression and Terminal Diseases**

Research has shown that people with low self-esteem are 32% more likely to die from cancer. Also, depression increases the chance of suffering from coronary disease. This claim is not farfetched because you'll not eat healthy meals when you're not in the right mental state. You'll not stick to a healthy plan by just eat whatever is available, which can have adverse effects on your physical health.

## Schizophrenia and Terminal Diseases

Experts have observed that schizophrenia patients are at double risk of dying from heart disease. They are also thrice at risk of dying from respiratory disease. This connection is because mental health patients aren't likely to receive routine checks such as weight, blood pressure, and cholesterol.

## Exercise and Depression

Research has proven that regular exercise affects the release and uptake of endorphins. These are chemicals in the brain that makes you feel happy. So, lack of exercise increases your chances of depression.

## Physical Exercise and Mental Alertness

Scientists have discovered that you can generate positive energy and improve your mental alertness through physical exercise. In fact, even a short burst of ten minutes fast walking can be a difference-maker.

# Doing It For Yourself

The advent of social media exposes us to multiple influences from various people across the world. It is easier to act in ways to fit into the crowd because you don't want to be rejected. This mindset can also affect your plan for a home workout. You might want to lose weight to earn the acceptance of people who don't care about you. This chapter reviews how to ensure you start on the right note by making your plan all about you.

## Avoiding Unnecessary Attention

The last thing you want is people paying attention to you unnecessarily because of your physique. Unfortunately, this is the experience of many people today, especially plus-size folks. The internet and movies are full of insensitive jokes to mock people because they are overweight. Indeed, it is not good to have excessive weight. It is not beneficial to your appearance, and it can also make you at risk of some health challenges, including obesity.

However, you shouldn't start your workout plan on the wrong note. There's nothing wrong with losing weight, but you shouldn't do so because you want to avoid unwarranted attention to yourself. Remember that developing muscle or losing weight is a gradual process. Of course, you should have a vision – a desired physique. Nonetheless, you need to learn to accept yourself while working towards your objective.

See yourself as someone who deserves the love and respect of other people regardless of your appearance. If you notice that your circle of friends often make insensitive comments about your looks, you

need to keep your distance from them. Be around people who aren't ashamed of you despite wanting you to get better.

Good friends will tell you your deficiencies and give you a roadmap to improve on them. They will support your plan and provide you with moral support to sustain your momentum. Besides, losing weight or building muscles does not mean that people will stop making jest of you. Insensitive people will always find reasons to mock you regardless of how successful you are. For example, Cristiano Ronaldo is one of the greatest footballers ever, but people still make demeaning remarks about him. So, learn to love and accept yourself regardless of your appearance.

# Keeping Fit With the Right Motive

In some fitness-based articles and books, the authors often encourage people to use negative comments and experiences as inspiration. For example, as a lady, if you were dumped by your boyfriend because you're overweight, they would encourage you to look sexy to get back at him. At the surface, it looks like a brilliant idea. You'll imagine going out on a date with another hot guy and posting the picture on social media. Nonetheless, it is a sign of insecurity.

Whoever breaks up with you because of your physique does not deserve your time. It is a different case if you have decided not to put in the effort to enhance your appearance. However, if a guy hooks up with another lady because he feels you're no longer as sexy as you used to be, he does not deserve you. It is the same for a lady who breaks up with a guy on the same grounds. The worst thing you can do is to start visiting the gym or starting a workout plan because of revenge.

If you start doing exercise to prove a point, you'll be frustrated and discouraged in the long run. Think about it; some guys still cheat on their spouse even when she is gorgeous. Many celebrities come to mind in this regard. In the same way, guys who have attractive abs lose their partners to other men. So, the issue is never because of physical appearance. If a person loves you, he or she will stick with you regardless of your physique. He or she might encourage you to lose weight, but it will never be by threatening to dump you for someone slimmer.

## Staying Clear of Media Pressure

Some people can recognize their source of stress. For example, you may know that your boss at work has been frustrating in recent times. In the same way, you may know that your kids or spouse have been making you unhappy recently. However, excessive exposure to media influences can affect you in ways you may never know. For example, you may be feeling bad about your body shape because of unpleasant comments after posting a picture.

Some people would post heavily edited pictures just to get likes and positive comments. Unfortunately, you might be feeling that such people have lives better than yourself. Meanwhile, they are just living a lie. Before you do anything, you need to ask yourself for the motive behind it. For example, you might want to start working out to earn more likes on social media. You might want to be given appellations such as hot, sexy, gorgeous, handsome, and the likes.

Indeed, such comments are nice and can put you in a good mood. However, it is a problem when you feel downtrodden or rejected because someone called you ugly or fat. You can become desperate and start working out to prove a point to such people. However, you'll not be able to sustain it. In fact, they can mock your effort to improve yourself.

Wait until you have the body shape you desire before posting videos or pictures if you want to inspire or encourage others. Don't post them to show to your detractors that you're making progress. They can laugh at you, and that will only affect your self-esteem further. You might need to take a break from the digital world to help put you back in charge of your life. This process is called digital detox. You can read "Disconnect to Reconnect" by the same author for more details.

## Signs You're Working Out For The Wrong Reasons

You can know when your motive for starting a workout is wrong. It will affect the way you go about it. The following symptoms shows that you need to review your motive or method:

- You're working out too hard due to impatience

- You're excessively indulging in one type of movement.

- Your body is overly sore with pain lingering for a week or more.

- You're feeling pain on one side of your body.

These signs are common to people who are trying to prove a point. You'll be fixated on one side of your body instead of overall health. Also, you'll be trying too hard because you're desperate.

# Benefits of Staying Fit

Understanding the benefits of an activity gives you the requisite impetus to sustain your momentum. Having a home workout plan offers you the following advantages.

## Prevents Muscle Loss

It's no news that your body will not function as efficiently as it used to as you grow older. Building muscles becomes more challenging, and the ones you have built will break down faster. Therefore, it is not shocking that older people look less attractive. They are like flowers that are gradually losing their beauty. The blossoms are eventually replaced by degradation.

You need to prepare for the latter periods of your life by having a plan for regular exercise. Nonetheless, you must go beyond just drawing out plans; you have to execute them. Regular exercise is an integral part of healthy aging. It helps you to maintain your muscle mass and also increase it. You might have seen people who still looked robust and active in their latter years. You can also be like that by working out.

Regular exercise keeps your metabolism high and gives you strength and resilience to complete your daily tasks. Indeed, you'll need the support of the people around you as you grow older. However, working out reduces your dependence on others. Moreover, it helps to prevent falling unconsciously, which is critical for older adults.

## Improves Digestion

Regular exercise is beneficial to your overall health, including digestion. When you have a culture of working out, you're doing your digestive tract a lot of good by strengthening it. Physical activities also keep the gut healthy. When you're less active, your intestinal flow becomes slower. Experts reckon that exercise has both short-term and long-term benefits.

It also alleviates gas, heartburn, constipation, and stomach cramps. Note that excessive or mistimed physical activities can have adverse effects on digestion. It can make you experience gastrointestinal problems such as abdominal pain, constipation, heartburn, bloating, and upset stomach. You can have these issues when you workout immediately after taking a meal. Therefore, exercise is beneficial to digestion when you do it before eating instead of after taking your meal.

Note that working out after eating is not always counterproductive. What matters is the timing. The reason working out is harmful immediately after taking your meal is that blood flows around your intestine and stomach to help with digestion. So, if you start exercising without allowing your body to rest, the blood will flow back to your stomach and other muscles, which could lead to digestion problems.

## Enhances Appearance

Working out improves your appearance in many ways. However, the two major ways it gives you a more youthful look is by building your muscles and improving your skin. Regular exercise detoxifies your skin of oils and dirt. How? Working out helps you to sweat more efficiently, which ensures that you lose toxins in your body through your skin pores.

So, with exercise, you might not need a detoxifying medication.

According to Audrey Kunin, a dermatologist in Kansas City, regular exercise is more like getting a mini-facial. She explained that working up a good sweat expels the sweat and oil trapped in your pores as they dilate. However, she recommends that you should ensure that you wash your face immediately you're done. Failure to do so will make the gunk get sucked back into your pores.

More so, regular exercise helps to relieve stress, which ensures that you look younger. Mental and physical exhaustion accelerates the aging process. Therefore, you give yourself a more youthful outlook by starting and sustaining your workout plan. Besides, building your muscles makes your clothes looked more fitted when you wear them, which improves your confidence when you step out.

# Improves Mental Performance and Work Productivity

You need to be calm and relaxed to succeed, especially when carrying out mentally taxing tasks. This state of mind is vital in the modern world where we work more with computers. So, to be at your best, you need to keep your focus whenever working. Meanwhile, one of the reasons you're distracted is because you aren't relaxed. Regular exercise offers you the requisite tranquility to excel in your daily activities.

With greater relaxation, comes enhanced efficiency. Remember that you cannot be at the apex of your career or fulfill your potential when you're fond of producing poor performances. Besides, there is a lot of pressure to perform or face the sack in the modern world because of its ultra-competitive nature. There are many people waiting in the wings to take your role and do a better job.

Even if you're an entrepreneur, you still need to be at the top of your game to stay relevant. The fierce competition of the business world requires that you're on your toes all the time. So, engaging in stress-relieving activities such as working out gives you a much- needed edge to have a clear mind.

# Have A New Circle of Productive Friends

You need positive energy around you to keep your sanity and fulfill your potential. It is imperative to keep the right company in a world of multiple negative influences. Many people out there are only interested in doing things that aren't productive, such as spending excessive time with digital devices or talking ill of others.

However, you can choose to rather spend your time doing things that can improve your health and performance. The truth is that you'll attract your kind. In other words, you'll easily make friends with people who share common interests with you. When you start working out, you'll mix up more with such people who like to invest their time in productive activities.

It is easier to meet these people when you join a health club. Note that the reason that making this move will make sense to you is that you're carrying out health-boosting activities. Working out makes you find other people doing the same thing. You'll share your improvements with them, and they can also give you tips that can make you more efficient.

# Viable Alternative to Social Media Activities

One of the best ways to curb a harmful habit is by replacing it with a positive one. For example, you may be addicted to a substance that improves your mood because you're often depressed. So, by having a hobby or doing sports, you might have more ways to make yourself happy instead of drug abuse.

In the same way, you might be addicted to digital devices because that is the only thing you do with your leisure period. However, you can break free from it by involving in productive activities such as visiting your loved ones or doing sports. Having a home workout plan is another helpful way to spend your time wisely because of the physical and mental health benefits it offers.

# The Science Behind Physical Fitness

According to Dr. Cheng, if the benefits of working out are put inside a drug, it would have been worth a million dollars. Researchers have always been interested in investigating the effects of regular exercise. The results have been promising. Here are some findings.

## Boosts the Immune System

A 2017 study revealed that a 20-minute moderate workout has tremendous effects on the immune system. The study involved 47 healthy volunteers. The participants were required to jog or walk on a treadmill, depending on their level of fitness. Before and after the exercise, the researchers measured an inflammatory marker's levels, TNF. They observed that there was a 5% reduction in the number of immune cells that generated the marker.

This result shows that physical activity could boost the immune system by preventing excessive inflammation. The researchers confirmed that working out has anti-inflammatory effects. Nonetheless, they were not able to explain the mechanism through which it takes place. Note that inflammation is a natural response of the immune system to injuries and diseases. However, when it is excessive, it can be counterproductive. It can lead to pain and other harmful effects.

Therefore, the fact that this study showed that exercise has anti- inflammatory effects is positive. It proves that it could protect you against chronic conditions due to moderate inflammatory responses. This result is liberating because it demonstrates that you might never have to invest in anti-inflammatory medications to rescue yourself from being at risk of excessive inflammatory responses. So, Dr. Cheng was right when he said that the advantages of working out are worth a million dollars.

## Reduces Cancer Risk

Cancer, in its various forms, is a devastating disease causing many people pain all over the world. Treating it can be challenging because it often requires surgery, which is expensive and also comes with various side effects. Therefore, prevention is the best approach when it comes to this ailment. The good news is that one of the ways you can reduce the risk of having cancer is by engaging yourself in regular exercise.

Studies have shown that routine physical activity is associated with reductions in the incidence of breast and colon cancer. A review of several studies demonstrated that moderate physical activity is linked with a greater protective effect than lesser intensity activities. The study showed that physically active men and women have a 30%–40% decrease in the risk of having colon cancer. The women, in particular, have a 20%–30% reduction in the risk of suffering from breast cancer.

The summary of this systematic review is that there is compelling evidence that working out is linked with a decrease in the prevalence of specific cancers. The authors believed people who engage in regular exercise are less likely to have breast and colon cancer, in particular. The researchers also confirmed that cancer patients who are involved in recreational physical activities are at a lower risk of dying of the disease when compared to those who are less active.

# Prevents Cardiovascular Disease

Generally, regular exercise boosts your heart rate, which bodes well for your overall health. Experts believe that women, in particular, have a lower chance of dying from specific diseases associated with physical inactivity. An example of such diseases is cardiovascular disease. Moreover, studies have proven that men and women who engage in regular exercise have a lesser risk of dying from heart- related illnesses.

For example, a study explored the effects of working out on the health of middle-aged men and women followed up for eight years. The researchers noticed that the lowest quintiles of physical fitness were associated with an increased risk of death from cardiovascular disease. Meanwhile, the top quintiles were linked to a decreased chance of mortality. Further research has only proven that the chances of dying from this disease are far less than earlier thought.

Recent investigations have demonstrated that being fit or active offers a greater than 50% reduction in the risk of death from heart-related sicknesses. These studies also showed that physically inactive middle-aged women experienced a 52% increase in all- cause mortality. These women engage in less than one hour of exercise per week. The scientists also confirmed that these people have a 29% increase in cancer-related mortality when compared to their physically active counterparts.

## Decreases Chances of Diabetes

Diabetes can be life-changing in a negative way. Apart from causing you agony, it will also prevent you from eating some of your favorite meals. However, scientists have discovered that you can protect yourself from suffering from this disease by engaging in regular workouts. For instance, a study revealed that both aerobic and resistance types of exercise are effective in preventing type 2 diabetes. The study involved 46 participants who are involved in energy-expending activities.

The researchers observed that regular exercise reduces the risk of type 2 diabetes by 6%. They noticed that this benefit was more

evident in people with a high body mass index. These participants are at higher risk of diabetes than the other participants.

Nonetheless, this study demonstrated that, apart from weight loss, working out also decreases the chances of becoming a diabetes patient. Several studies have supported this investigation, proving that the findings are reliable.

For example, a study involving 271 male physicians recorded similar results. The research showed that the participants who reported weekly physical activity had a reduced incidence of type 2 diabetes. The activities they carried out were sufficient to make them sweat. The researchers explained that these participants also have a lesser chance of battling cardiovascular ailment.

## Improves Bone Health

If you want to improve your bone density, you need to have a culture of regular workout. Weight-bearing exercise, particularly resistance exercise, has the most effects on bone mineral density. A review of several cross-sectional reports proved that doing resistance training increases bone mineral density. Therefore,
those that engage in these activities have a

higher chance of having healthier bones than those that don't do them.

More so, the authors observed that the type of sports you engage in determines your bone mineral density. For example, athletes who participate in low-impact sports tend to have lower bone mineral density when compared with athletes who are involved in high- impact sports. Therefore, although working out improves bone health, some specific routines have significant impacts than others. Other researchers have gotten similar results in studies involving children, adolescents, middle-aged and older adults.

Numerous longitudinal studies have examined the effects of exercise on bone health using various categories of people. The scientists recommend that more studies are needed, especially the ones involving more participants. Nonetheless, the studies so far have shown that there is compelling proof that physical activities improve bone health. They also reduce the chance of suffering from bone-related diseases. Researchers suggest that weight-bearing and impact exercise enables you to avoid bone loss associated with aging.

# Physical Fitness and Your Sex Life

Regular exercise has a plethora of benefits, as you have seen through the science-based evidence in the previous chapter. So, you have more than enough reasons to start and sustain a workout plan. Nevertheless, physical fitness also helps you in your sex life.

Indeed, you shouldn't be involved in exercise solely for the sake of boosting your sexual prowess and adventures. However, we cannot deny that physical fitness goes a long way in helping you in this aspect. This chapter reviews the link between staying fit and your sex life.

## Attracting the Opposite Sex

It is true that what many people find attractive in the long run defers. Some people find brilliant people attractive, while some people find emotionally intelligent people appealing. Nonetheless,

the reality is that the outward appearance often encourages you to check inside the "container." One of the worst kept secrets in the world is that people are moved by what they see. Humans tend to believe that good-looking people can do no wrong until they do so.

Indeed, you want people to see the qualities beyond your appearance. However, you need to help them by looking good. You may have fantastic traits that will make you an excellent romantic partner and still struggle to find a spouse because of the way you look. Only a few people are patient and insightful enough to look
beyond the surface. So, you need to do your part to give yourself a higher chance of meeting the man or woman of your dream.

You should be able to look at yourself in the mirror and smile because of your physique. If you're objective enough, you might admit that you'll not want to date yourself if you were the opposite sex. Therefore, start your workout plan to give yourself that admirable figure. Remember that this shouldn't be your main focus for involving in regular exercise. Nonetheless, it is an added advantage that can make a significant difference.

# Self-Confidence When Asking or Going For A Date

Confidence is a vital trait that helps you to achieve remarkable success in every aspect, including your sex life. If you have low self-esteem, people that are less qualified for a role will be selected ahead of you. Everyone wants to be with someone they can trust to handle a job. Indeed, some people can be overconfident such that they promise what they cannot offer. However, such people will

always get opportunities to prove themselves more than people who have low self-confidence.

When it comes to relating with the opposite sex, you need to be assured to get a date. Also, you need high self-esteem to cope with the eventualities of going out on a date. When you aren't self- confident, you can make silly mistakes that are very avoidable. In the movie "Aladdin," the main character ruined his first opportunity to impress the princess because he was anxious. He said things he had to apologize for later because he was not assured in himself.

Meanwhile, having a good appearance gives you the requisite confidence to apply yourself appropriately when speaking to the opposite sex. You love to have that body shape any man or woman will desire. This confidence also goes into the bedroom. When you have a great physique, you'll want to show it off to your partner, and this affects your performance.

# Keeping Fit and Libido

Physical activity has multiple effects on functioning during sex. It can be positive or negative, depending on how you go about it. According to a study by the University of California, men who involve in regular exercise have significantly enhanced performance during sex. They also have a higher percentage of satisfying orgasms. This study also showed that women who are physically active enjoy the same perks.

A study by the University of Texas also investigated the link between physical fitness and sexual performance. The researchers observed that working out boosts physiological sexual arousal in women. This result shows that ladies who engage in exercise are more likely to be turned on than those who don't.

Experts believe that physical activity plays a vital role in sexual performance because it increases breathing, heart rate, and muscular activity. This enhancement ultimately affects sexual performance and sexual satisfaction.

Nonetheless, you need to tread carefully. You can ruin your sex life when you excessively exert yourself during workouts. Research has found out that men who involve in strenuous exercise on a regular
basis could have significantly decreased libido. This study was carried out by scientists from the University of North Carolina at Chapel Hill. In other words, men who engage in lower-intensity exercise could have better sex performance than their higher- intensity counterparts.

# Fatigue, Mental Exhaustion, and Sex

There are different ways your body can react when you're stressed. One of them is that it can sabotage your workout. Besides, your libido can also suffer. Stress increases the production of a hormone called cortisol, which can reduce your interest in sex in the long run.

Meanwhile, exercise produces the feel-good hormone, endorphins, which lower cortisol levels.

Lower cortisol levels will, in turn, reduce your stress levels and boost your sexual arousal. Therefore, working out enhances your sex drive. According to Dr. Penhollow, physical activity reduces depression. Meanwhile, you aren't likely to have sexual desires when you aren't in a good mood. So, by reducing or eliminating
depression, regular exercise enhances your sex life by boosting your sex drive.

Additionally, working out improves your flexibility, which boosts your ability to try different sex positions that are more satisfying. Moreover, you need body strength to hold or sustain some sexual moves. Therefore, by involving in regular exercise, you'll give yourself the vitality and power needed to engage in optimum sexual activity.

## Sex-boosting Exercises

The following activities, in particular, can boost your sexual performance:

## Kegels

Kegels exercises strengthen pelvic floor muscles. Therefore, experts believe that it could help enhance libido in both men and women. These exercises are also recommended to alleviate problems with bowel control or urine leakage. In women, these activities could

strengthen vaginal muscles, which promote a more powerful orgasm. It could also help delay ejaculation in men.

## Strength Training

This exercise involves using weights or resistance to make your muscles stronger. Experts reckon that this type of workout is better than cardio exercises such as walking a treadmill when it comes to relieving stress.

## Walking

Walking for just thirty minutes around your house can make a tremendous impact on your overall health. Specifically, it can decrease the risk of suffering erectile dysfunction in men. A Harvard study revealed that it reduces the chance of erectile dysfunction by 41%.

# Swimming

You may not be able to swim every day, unlike walking. Nonetheless, just thirty minutes of this activity three times a week

can boost your sex drive according to the same study. It can also lead to weight loss, which enhances sexual sustenance.

# Tips on Creating a Feasible Workout Plan

Working out at home comes with a lot of advantages. You'll not have to spend money transporting yourself to and from the gym. It also affords you the time for a thorough warm-up before starting a session. Meanwhile, with some minutes of warming up, you're ready to fire on all cylinders. It is not ideal to start a session with cold muscles to avoid injuries during the activity. This chapter will guide you through how to create your own home workout plan.

## Crescendo all the way: Starting with the Easiest Tasks

Remember that desperation will only get you undesirable results. Therefore, when starting your home workout, you need to set clearly defined goals to channel your energy in the right direction. You should ask yourself the following questions and many more:

- Do I want to lose weight?

- Am I trying to bulk up or build muscle?

Regardless of your reason for involving in regular exercise, you should start from the easiest tasks. Write down your targets so that they can serve as inspiration and motivation later. Nonetheless, you need to take it slowly to avoid getting injuries or overstretching your muscles.

# Typical Home Workout Plan

Your objectives will determine your home workout plan. You can do more research regarding specific exercises that favor your goals. As a beginner, you can choose to start by working out three days a week. If you're choosing Mondays, Wednesdays, and Fridays, a typical week's routine looks like this:

# Workout 1: Monday

After warming up for a few minutes, you can start your routine with the following activities:

## Activity #1 Power Snatch

This exercise involves bending your knees while holding a dumbbell in one hand between your legs. Then extend your hips, knees, and ankles explosively to raise the weight overhead. Drop into a half squat to hold the weight overhead once your body is straight from head to toe, then stand up straight. It is recommended that you rest for a minute before moving to the next activity.

## Activity #2 Squat Press

Begin with the dumbbells at shoulder level and go down into a squat. Proceed by standing up and press the weights directly overhead. Bring down the weights and go back to the initial position.

## Activity #3 Jump Squat

After resting for sixty seconds, start with the dumbbells by your sides, and go down into a half squat. Then jump straight up from the ground, land softly, and do it again.

### Activity #4 Windmill

Begin by holding a dumbbell overhead before bending at the waist by bringing one hand down your leg. Ensure that you focus on the weight throughout the routine.

### Activity #5 Roll-Out

With the dumbbells below your shoulders, kneel. Then roll the weights forwards as far as possible. Control the movement with

your abs, then return to the initial position. This move, alongside windmill, is the best way to develop a rock-hard six-pack.

# Workout 2: Wednesday

Just like the first day, focus more on functional movements. These activities aren't difficult and give you the momentum to keep going when you're beginning to tire out. They include dumbbell swing, overhead squat, side lunge, press-up renegade row, and leg raise. Make the exercise seamless by resting for a minute after completing a task.

## Activity #1 Dumbbell Swing

By hinging at the hips, send the dumbbell between your legs. Then in order to use the hip drive to raise the dumbbell to shoulder height, push your glutes forwards powerfully. Reverse the move to the beginning and move to the next rep.

## Activity #2 Overhead Squat

This activity involves starting with both holding the weights directly overhead. Then bend at the hips and knees to lower into a squat at the same time. Ensure that you don't allow the weights to come forward.

## Activity #3 Press-Up Renegade Row

Perform a press-up at the top while holding a dumbbell in each hand. Ensure you row one dumbbell up to your side. Then row the other dumbbell up while lowering the weight to complete one rep.

## Activity #4 Side Lunge

Begin by holding a dumbbell in each hand. Then bend your leading knee as you take a big step to one side. Make sure that you keep your foot pointing forwards while your knee is in line with your toes. Return to the start by pushing off your leading foot. Then take move other way to repeat the movement. With each rep, alternate sides.

## Activity #5 Leg Raise

This exercise is quite straightforward. It involves holding a dumbbell between your feet with your heels elevated slightly off the ground. Raise your legs until they are vertical while keeping them straight. Then slowly lower under control while ensuring that your heels don't touch the floor.

# Workout 3: Friday

In the last workout day of the week, it is recommended that you end on a high. In other words, do more tedious tasks. In this routine, the first one here might be the most challenging exercise you have ever attempted. The issue is not complexity or heaviness, but technicality. Pressing weights directly overhead while squatting demands excellent mobility and control. The last activity is the Turkish get-ups. This activity is so demanding and beneficial that you can make it an entire session.

### Activity #1 Back of Steel

Start by lowering into an overhead squat with the dumbbells above your head. Then lower the weights to shoulder level while still in a squat position. Continue by repeating the lowering and pressing movement while in the position.

### Activity #2 One-Leg Squat

With the dumbbells by your sides, stand on one leg. Then bend at the hips and knees to lower into a single-leg squat while keeping your chest up. Press back up to where you began. Endeavor to complete all the reps on that leg before switching to the other.

### Activity #3 Woodchop Lunge

Start this exercise by placing a dumbbell over a shoulder. Then lunge forwards with the opposite leg while bringing the weight down across your body at the same time. Swap sides after doing all the reps on one side.

## Activity #4 One-Leg Romanian Deadlift

With the weights hanging down by your thighs, stand on one leg. Lower the weights towards the floor by hinging at the hips. Ensure that you keep them close to your leg. You'll put a strain on your lower back if you come too far forward. So, avoid it.

## Activity #5 Turkish Get-Up

End the session by lying on the floor as you hold a weight above your face. Then bend your knee on that side and come up onto your elbow. Move to your hand and push your hips off the floor. Then bring your straight leg back under your body. Remove your hand from the floor and stand up.

# How To Create A Diet Plan

You cannot have an effective workout plan without an equally excellent diet plan. Exercise is a physical activity, and you need the energy to make it work. Besides, a good eating habit by itself affects your appearance. Therefore, it is imperative that you have a healthy eating habit to ensure that your effort is not futile. This chapter examines the right way to go about creating a diet plan that will complement your workout plan.

## The Link Between Physical Fitness and Feeding Habits

Physical activity requires "fuel" to make it run smoothly. Therefore, the relevance of food to your workout plan cannot be overemphasized. When you start engaging in exercise, you'll be fitter and lose weight. Nonetheless, your energy needs will also change. You'll need more calories to keep up with the metabolism and activities going on in your body. You'll need an adequate amount of the following as a physically active individual:

- Carbohydrates, which is the body's primary source of energy.

- Fat, which is an additional source of vitality.

- Protein, which is vital to the maintenance and rebuild of tissues, including muscles.
- Water, which is critical to the replacement of fluids lost during the activity.

In order to have these essential nutrients, you need to eat a moderate, varied, and balanced diet. Too much or too little of them will not aid your objective of giving your body what it needs to support and sustain your workout plan. Moderate implies that you should eat a little of everything without anything in excess. It is possible to have every essential class of food in your food without eating too much.

Varied means that while eating different food types, you'll still ensure that you always get the nutrients you need. In other words, you'll eat other fruits instead of just apple, for example. Note that no one food provides any particular nutrient. So, eat a wide variety of food to avoid overeating any substance, which will not be beneficial to your body. Meanwhile, balanced implies that you'll eat the recommended number of servings from each food type most days.

Athletes and people who are very physically active have special nutritional requirements because of the demands they place on their bodies. They often need more carbohydrates like grains more than the amount required by an average person. However, they don't need as much protein as other people.

The liver and muscles store carbohydrates as ready energy, and this supply is rapidly consumed during exercise. Endurance athletes such as cyclists and runners require a large amount of this nutrient because of the nature of their activities. They need to eat the carbohydrate before or during the exercise because the body does not have the capacity to store a lot of it.

## Typical Diet Plan

The scope of this book covers a two weeks diet plan that is scientifically designed for substantial weight loss. It offers approximately 1250 calories daily, which is more than enough for a physically active individual. Below is a summary of the basic dietary guidelines.

It outlines the daily amount of food that is permitted from each food class. Endeavor to mix and match food items all day long. Make sure that you don't exceed your caloric goal while doing this. You can follow one of the pre-designed menus below to ensure that you're doing the right thing.

# Nutrition Guidelines

Vegetables: One and a half cups (half cup is equivalent to: half cup of raw/cooked/frozen/canned veggies, one cup of leafy greens, or half cup vegetable juice). Pick different options, which can include starchy veggies, orange veggies, dry beans, dark green veggies, and peas.

Oils: Four teaspoons (one teaspoon is equivalent to: one teaspoon vegetable oil, two teaspoons light salad dressing, one teaspoon butter, or one teaspoon of low- fat mayo).

Fruit: One cup (one cup is equivalent to: one cup of frozen/fresh/ canned fruits, half cup dried fruits, or one cup fruit juices). Healthy choices include pears, apples, mangoes, cherries, grapes, raspberries, strawberries, blueberries, and pomegranates.

Grains: Four ounces (one ounce is equivalent to: one slice bread, one cup of cereal flakes, one small muffin, half cup cooked rice, or one ounce dry pasta).

Milk: Two cups (one cup is equivalent to: one cup of yogurt/milk/ soy milk or one and a half ounces of cheese. Choose low-fat or non- fat options as much as possible.

Meats and Beans: Three ounces (One ounce is equivalent to: One ounce lean poultry/meat/ fish, one egg, one tablespoon peanut butter, quarter cup cooked beans, or half ounce nuts/seeds).

**Menu #1**

**Breakfast (8 am – 9 am)**

One slice of toast

Smoothie (blend one cup soymilk and ice cubes + one cup berries together)
One teaspoon of butter

## Lunch (11 am – 1 pm)

There-quarter cup vegetables (such as carrots, steamed broccoli, cauliflower, etc.) One cup cooked grain (such as brown rice, white rice, wild rice, millet, quinoa, etc.) Two ounces of lean meat (around the size of half deck of playing cards) Snack (3pm – 4pm)

A half ounce of seeds or one egg

## Dinner (5 pm – 7 pm)

Two teaspoons light dressing

One and a half cups of leafy greens One and a half ounces of cheese

## Menu #2

## Breakfast (8 am – 9 am)

One cup of yogurt A Half cup oatmeal Herbal tea or black coffee

## Lunch (11 am – 1 pm)

One slice whole wheat bread

Tomato, cucumber, lettuce (equivalent to three-quarter cup total) Two ounces of tuna
One teaspoon olive oil +
one teaspoon mayo
Snack (3 pm – 4 pm)
One piece of fruit or one cup of fresh fruit or

## Dinner (5 pm – 7 pm)

One corn tortilla

Half cup shredded lettuce Half cup salsa
Half cup black beans One half ounce cheese
Half cup cooked rice

## Menu #3

## Breakfast (8 am – 9 am)

Half cup milk/soy milk One cup high fiber
cereal One banana

## Lunch (11 am – 1 pm)

One cup raw carrot
sticks/celery/green peppers
One cup of pasta
Two teaspoons of olive oil Two ounces of lean
meat Snack (3 pm – 4 pm)
Half cup vegetables or half cup pasta sauce

## Dinner (5 pm – 7 pm)

One cup low-fat cottage cheese Six crackers Half ounce mixed nuts

# Tips for Dieting Success

Following a strict diet plan is easier said than done. Nonetheless, the following hints can help you succeed in this endeavor:

- Plan for every week ahead of time.

- Clear your fridge and pantry of every food item that can potentially derail your diet plan. This is an easy way to avoid temptations.

- Consume eight or more glasses of water daily. Also, drink at least a glass before every meal to avoid overeating by decreasing your appetite.

- It takes around twenty minutes before your brain notifies you that you're full. Therefore, eat slowly as much as possible. Chew each bite and put your fork or spoon down between bites.

- Bring variety to an otherwise restricted diet by trying new foods whenever possible.

- Increase your chances of feeling satisfied by adding spices to your food for flavor.

- Resist the urge of to eat excessively outside by cooking for yourself.

- In order to avoid being tempted to take a snack after a meal, brush your teeth. Lack of sleep can stimulate appetite and lead to overeating. So, get adequate sleep.
- Most importantly, never forget your objective.

# How To Maintain Your Plan and Momentum

It is easy to start anything, but it can be challenging to stick with a plan and accomplish the goal. You can draft a diet and workout plan after reading this book. Nonetheless, you'll find reasons to stop over time. There will be days when you're discouraged and don't feel like continuing again. However, you can ensure that you retain your focus and maintain your consistency by leveraging the following tips.

## Be Consistent with Time and Location

When you carry out an activity, it is an act. However, when you carry it out regularly, it becomes a habit. Note that you can train your body in such a way that you'll crave to do something all over again. It is possible to do something repeatedly in such a way that you'll feel like something is missing whenever you didn't do it.

Examples of such daily tasks we train ourselves to do daily include brushing the teeth and taking your bath.

In some cases, you can feel like your life is out of place whenever you didn't carry out these tasks. You can train your body to see your home workout plan that way. The key to making this possible is to be consistent with time and venue. Avoid using different places and periods as much as possible. When you do something at a particular time during a particular day at a specific location, your body will get used to it.

You'll desire to do it again whenever that time gets closer. You may need an alarm at the early stage. However, after a week or two of consistent workout, your body will be used to it. Your body will have a natural timer that reminds you that it is getting close to that period. Even if you forget to carry out the activity, you'll still remember later in the day because it has become part and parcel of your daily tasks.

# Always Remind Yourself About the Benefits

There is no point in doing something without doing it well. Meanwhile, you cannot enjoy the benefits of carrying out an activity without doing it consistently, and workout is no different. You cannot get that body shape you desire when you're unstable in the way you go about your exercise. Also, you cannot lose weight or build your muscles to your taste when you aren't consistent. Therefore, you need to retain your focus on the advantages to spur yourself to keep going.

Write out your goals from onset to make it easier for you to keep remembering them. You can make them a note reminder in short forms on your phone. Besides, you can also make them short notes and place them in conspicuous places in your house to remind you. You have to leverage your environment to set yourself up to succeed in your plan. For example, if you use a mat during your exercise, you can spread it close to your bed before you sleep to remind yourself the following morning.

These are just examples. Think about other

creative ways you can help yourself to remember to stick to your plan. Only those that sustain the initial momentum and motivation will achieve their

targets. Note that being motivated is not enough because there will be days when your passion will be low. Nonetheless, by reminding yourself about what you need to achieve, you'll be able to inspire yourself to stay committed.

## Surround Yourself with the Right People

The importance of having the right people around you cannot be overemphasized. Determination is the most critical ingredient that will see you succeed in any task. However, it is possible that you lose your initial zeal when you have people around you that don't value what you're doing. They will tell you that you're just making yourself go through unnecessary stress. They might even point out studies such as the one cited earlier about strenuous exercise leading to a reduction in libido.

Note that you don't need the right people around you for the good days when you're motivated. When you're zealous about something, it is difficult for anyone to convince you otherwise. Nevertheless, the problem is that you'll not always be passionate. In fact, there might be days when you mistakenly injure yourself

while carrying out a physical activity. A circumstance like this can discourage you from engaging in regular workouts.

It is during those days when you aren't inspired to continue again that you need the right people that can encourage you. They will remind you about your goals and help you get back to your feet again. Remember that you're working out at home. So, you may not have access to such people physically. However, you can meet them by joining a group or page on social media where people share their experiences, challenges, and victories.

# Keep A Journal of Your Progress

Having a culture of keeping a journal offers a variety of advantages. One of them is that it enables you to keep your thoughts organized. It enables you to record daily thoughts, feelings, and events. If you want to train your writing, keeping a journal is one of the ways to do it. You'll learn to write a specific topic and develop your ideas, thereby improving your writing skills. However, journaling is a veritable tool that can help you achieve your goals.

Your journal is the best place to highlight your goals, including your workout objectives. Anytime you need to update it, you'll remember the targets again and have renewed optimism and commitment to follow through on your plan. Besides, it is a convenient and practical way to monitor your progress. Whenever you record your milestones, you'll be excited to keep going. You can highlight the next target and how you intend to achieve it.

Additionally, keeping a journal enables you to record ideas on the go. You can jot down new tips that can help you improve or stick with your diet and workout plan. You'll not be limited by location or time when you have a journal. Besides, updating your journal helps you relieve stress. You can write down your anxieties and

frustrations there instead of keeping them on your mind. This approach helps you to improve your overall health by releasing tension.

## Share Your Results with People of Like Minds

Talking about something shows your conviction about it. Besides, the more you discuss an idea, the sounder you'll be about it. So, it is vital to share your plans, experiences, and improvements with other people to keep you interested and motivated. Nonetheless, you should be careful about the kind of individuals you talk to about your workout plan. From your previous interactions, you can know people who aren't likely to share a common interest with you.

If you talk to people who don't value exercise, they might discourage you. As mentioned earlier, if you cannot find people around you that are also fascinated and enthusiastic about engaging in exercise, you can join a page or group on social media to that effect. You'll find many individuals who are at the same level and those who at advanced stages. You'll learn from their mistakes and disappointments to improve your routine.

Such avenues also provide you with the opportunity to share your experiences and shortcomings with other people. You'll easily find tips and hints that can help you improve. You'll realize that there are other people that are also experiencing the same struggles. If you have questions, you'll be able to ask them, and you'll find helpful answers that can help you improve your plan. Whenever you reach a milestone, such platforms afford you the opportunity to share your happiness with people of like passion.

# Conclusion

The most limiting factor when it comes to achieving a target is a lack of quality information. Nonetheless, knowledge is not enough to succeed in any endeavor. You need to be committed to implementing the ideas you have received to record remarkable success. Reading this book has given you the information required to create and sustain an effective home workout plan. However, if you don't implement the ideas, the knowledge is pointless.

So, do more than get vital tips for your regular exercise. Ensure that you follow up on the knowledge by using it. You have been taught to write out your goals for your workout plan. However, there are many other benefits that you can enjoy apart from your objectives. Many of them have been mentioned earlier.

They include improved sleep, stress relief, depression reduction, and a decrease in cancer and diabetes risk. The advantages are science-based facts. Therefore, starting and sticking with your workout plan is one of the best decisions you can make.

You can still get the body shape you desire that will give you the requisite confidence to excel in different aspects of your life. Also, you can stay fit to improve your sexual performance to your partner's satisfaction. You can also avoid attracting unwanted attention to yourself and being ridiculed because of your weight. Nothing can stop you if you are determined. Begin your workout and diet plan today to give yourself a new lease of life.

CPSIA information can be obtained
at www.ICGtesting.com
Printed in the USA
LVHW111640310121
677958LV00015B/147